HOW TO FIX SLEEP PROBLEMS

PROFESSIONAL REMEDIES FOR SLEEP PROBLEMS

A.D RAMS

Contents

CHAPTER ONE

INTRODUCTION

Our everyday lives depend on sleep because it affects our physical and mental health as well as our overall productivity. On the other hand, getting a good night's sleep might be difficult for a lot of people. Difficulties with falling asleep, staying asleep, or having poor quality sleep can all have a big influence on our life.

We will go over a number of methods and approaches in this extensive guide to assist you in regaining control over your sleep health and overcoming sleep issues. This article tries to offer doable methods for enhancing your sleep quality, from comprehending the significance of sleep hygiene to putting relaxation techniques into practice and investigating any underlying problems.

We'll explore the science of sleep, identify common sleep problems, and talk about lifestyle changes that can improve your sleep quality. We'll also talk about how technology, food, and surroundings may all help you develop healthier sleeping patterns.

You will have a toolset of techniques at your disposal to successfully manage your sleep issues by the time you finish reading this guide. The information in this article will enable you to make significant adjustments and establish a more restorative sleep schedule, regardless of whether you're trying to improve the quality of your sleep or are dealing with insomnia or sleep apnea.

Recall that enhancing the quality of your sleep is a journey that calls for perseverance, consistency, and an openness to trying out new strategies. Through commitment and appropriate education, you may conquer sleep issues and get the numerous advantages of restorative sleep.

Comprehending the Significance of Sleep

One of the most important physiological processes for general health and wellbeing is sleep. It is a recurrent, naturally occurring state of diminished consciousness and reactivity to outside stimuli. Even if the precise purposes of sleep are still unknown, studies have shown that sleep is crucial to many aspects of our existence. These include:

Rest and Rejuvenation: Sleep enables the body to heal and regenerate. The body goes through processes that include tissue healing, memory consolidation, and regulation of several bodily functions while you sleep.

Memory Consolidation: Sleep is essential for fortifying and preserving memories that were created while awake. Better learning and memory retention result from the brain processing and storing information learned during the day while you sleep.

Cognitive Function: For the best possible attention, focus, problem-solving, and decision-making, getting enough sleep is crucial. Prolonged sleep deprivation can damage key brain functions, resulting in worse performance and productivity.

Emotional Control: Sleep is essential for controlling feelings and mood. Sleep deficiency can cause irritation, mood fluctuations, and increased emotional reactivity, whereas getting enough sleep promotes emotional stability and resilience.

Physical Health: Getting enough sleep is essential for sustaining a strong immune system, controlling hunger and metabolism, and promoting cardiovascular health. Chronic sleep deprivation has been linked to a higher risk of developing heart disease, diabetes, obesity, impaired immunological function, and weakened cardiac function.

Hormonal Regulation: The hormones that control growth, hunger, metabolism, and stress response are secreted in response to sleep. Hormone imbalances brought on by sleep disturbances might have an impact on one's general health and wellbeing.

Brain Health: For general mental well-being and cognitive performance, getting enough sleep is crucial. Sleep promotes optimal brain function and lowers the risk of neurodegenerative disorders like Alzheimer's disease by removing waste products and poisons from the brain.

Despite how important sleep is, a lot of individuals have trouble getting enough or high-quality sleep because of a variety of things, including stress, lifestyle decisions, illnesses, and sleep disorders. Making good sleep hygiene practices a priority can help increase the quantity and quality of sleep, which can enhance general health and wellbeing. These activities include adhering to a regular sleep schedule, setting up a pleasant sleeping environment, and learning relaxing techniques.

Recognizing Typical Sleep Issues

People may encounter a number of common sleep issues at some point in their lives. The quality of sleep, general health, and day-to-day functioning can all be severely impacted by these sleep disorders. Among the most typical issues with sleep are:

The inability to fall asleep, stay asleep, or wake up too early and not be able to go back to sleep are the symptoms of insomnia. Numerous things, such as stress, worry, sadness, irregular sleeping patterns, or underlying medical disorders, might contribute to it.

The disorder known as sleep apnea is characterized by shallow or periodic breathing while you sleep. It may result in additional health issues, excessive daytime sleepiness, and disturbed sleep. The two primary forms of sleep apnea are central sleep apnea (CSA), in which the brain fails to deliver signals to the muscles controlling breathing, and obstructive sleep apnea (OSA), in which the airway gets clogged during sleep.

The neurological condition known as restless legs syndrome (RLS) is typified by painful feelings in the legs that are frequently described as crawling, tingling, itching, or creeping. These feelings might make it difficult to fall or remain asleep at night and usually get worse at that time.

Periodic Limb Movement Disorder (PLMD): This condition causes the arms or legs to move repeatedly and uncontrollably as you sleep, which can cause frequent awakenings or disturbed sleep. These can be more marked jerking actions or more subdued twitches.

Hypersomnia during the day, abrupt episodes of muscle weakness or paralysis (cataplexy), vivid hallucinations during sleep or wakefulness (hypnagogic or hypnopompic hallucinations), and disturbed sleep at night are the hallmarks of narcolepsy, a neurological condition.

Parasomnias: During sleep, strange movements or actions take place. Night terrors, sleepwalking, sleep talking, and REM sleep behavior disorder (RBD), in which people act out their dreams, are a few examples.

A person with shift work sleep disorder experiences difficulties sleeping at desired times and excessive drowsiness or sleeplessness during work hours. This condition is caused by a conflict between the person's work schedule and their natural sleep-wake cycle.

Disorders of the Circadian Rhythm: These conditions cause irregularities in the body's internal clock, which affect the sleep-wake cycle. Jet lag, advanced sleep phase disorder (ASPD), and delayed sleep phase disorder (DSPD) are a few examples.

It is essential to recognize and treat these sleep issues in order to enhance the quality of sleep, general health, and functioning during the day. Speaking with a medical expert, such as a primary care physician or sleep specialist, can assist in identifying underlying sleep issues and creating a personalized treatment plan. Treatments for sleep apnea may involve behavioral therapy, drugs, lifestyle changes, or treatments like continuous positive airway pressure (CPAP) therapy.

Evaluating Sleep Patterns and Habits

Evaluating sleep patterns and routines is crucial to spotting possible problems that could be compromising overall health and the quality of sleep. When evaluating sleep patterns and behaviors, take into account the following actions and inquiries:

Sleep Routine:

What time do you usually wake up on the weekends and what time do you go to bed?

Do you sleep at around the same hours every day, or do you vary greatly from day to day?

Can you obtain adequate sleep every night to feel refreshed and focused during the day?

Ambience for Sleep:

Is it comfortable to sleep in your bedroom? Is everything cozy, calm, and dark?

Do you have any noise, light, or uncomfortable temperature disturbances in your bedroom that could be interfering with your sleep?

How close to bedtime do you use electronic devices (such as computers, tablets, and cellphones) before going to bed?

CHAPTER TWO

Quality of Sleep:

On an average night, how would you rank the quality of your sleep? When you wake up, do you feel rested and alert, or do you feel exhausted and foggy?

Do you have trouble falling asleep at night or remaining asleep throughout the day?

Do you often wake up throughout the night, and if so, do you find it difficult to go back to sleep?

Suitable Sleep Position:

What sleep-related rituals or habits do you have? Do you read a book or take a warm bath before going to bed to unwind?

If you drink alcohol, smoke, or take caffeine right before bed, how does it impact your sleep?

If you work out on a regular basis, when do you work it out earlier in the day or right before bed?

During the day:

Do you feel too tired or sleepy during the day?

Do you find it hard to focus during the day, to recall things, or to stay awake?

Have your mood or irritation changed in any way that you might associate with your sleeping patterns?

Health Background and Medications:

Do you suffer from any underlying medical ailments that could interfere with your ability to sleep, such as mental health issues, respiratory issues, or chronic pain?

Do you now take any medications that could affect how well or how often you sleep?

Disorders of Sleep:

Have you ever received a diagnosis for narcolepsy, sleep apnea, insomnia, or restless legs syndrome?

Do you have any symptoms, such loud snoring, gasping for air while you sleep, or abrupt paralysis or weakness of the muscles during the day, that point to a sleep disorder?

Individuals and healthcare providers can obtain important insights into potential sleep-related problems and create individualized plans for enhancing sleep quality and general well-being by carefully evaluating various components of sleep patterns and behaviors.

Establishing a Sleep-Friendly Space

Establishing a sleep-friendly atmosphere is crucial for encouraging deep, restful sleep. The following advice will help you optimize your bedroom and surroundings to enhance the quality of your sleep:

Darkness: Use blackout curtains or shutters to block out outside light sources in order to create the darkest possible environment in your bedroom. If eliminating all sources of light is not possible, think about using an eye mask.

Quietness: To reduce disturbing noises, use earplugs, a white noise machine, or relaxing sounds like nature sounds or peaceful music.

pleasant Temperature: To encourage sleep, keep your room at a pleasant temperature, usually between 60 and 67 degrees Fahrenheit (15 and 20 degrees Celsius). To get the perfect temperature for you, turn on your thermostat or cover up with blankets as necessary.

Comfy Bedding: Make an investment in pillows and a comfy mattress that will support your body well. Select bedding that is breathable, such linen or cotton, to assist maintain comfort and help control body temperature.

Clutter-Free Ambience: To establish a tranquil and soothing ambiance that promotes restful sleep, keep your bedroom tidy, orderly, and clutter-free. Take out all work-related documents, electronics, and other distractions from your bedroom.

Limit Screen Time: Steer clear of using electronics like computers, televisions, tablets, and cellphones right before bed since the blue light they generate might disrupt the body's natural production of melatonin, a hormone that controls sleep-wake cycles.

Establish a Calm Routine: To let your body know when it's time to wind down and get ready for sleep, create a calm routine for bedtime. This could involve doing things like reading, having a warm bath, meditating, or deep breathing, or just listening to relaxing music.

Limit Stimulants: Refrain from drinking stimulants such as alcohol, nicotine, and coffee right before bed because they can interfere with your ability to fall asleep and stay asleep all night.

Reduce Daytime Napping: If you struggle to fall asleep at night, try cutting down on or eliminating daytime naps, especially in the late afternoon or evening, as they may make it more difficult for you to doze off at night.

Frequent Exercise: Get moving during the day, but steer clear of intense exercise right before bed as this might heighten alertness and complicate falling asleep. To encourage higher-quality sleep, try to do some moderate activity in early in the day.

You may maximize the amount of peaceful, revitalizing sleep that you get by putting these tips into practice and making your bedroom and surroundings sleep-friendly.

Adopting Good Sleep Habits

Adopting routines and actions that support adequate sleep quantity and quality is part of practicing proper sleep hygiene. The following are essential pointers for creating a restful sleep schedule:

Keep a Regular Sleep Schedule: Even on weekends, go to bed and wake up at the same time every day. Maintaining consistency improves the quality of your sleep and aids your body's internal clock.

Establish a Calm Before Bedtime habit: Set up a peaceful habit that helps your body know when it's time to relax and go to sleep. This could be doing relaxation techniques, reading, having a warm bath, or listening to calming music.

Establish a Comfortable Sleep Environment: Keep your bedroom cold, dark, and quiet to promote restful sleep. Invest in cozy bedding, block off light with blackout curtains or blinds, and, if needed, use a white noise machine or earplugs to drown out noisy neighbors.

Reduce Screen Time Before Bed: Give yourself at least an hour's notice before going to bed to avoid using electronics like TVs, laptops, tablets, and smartphones. These gadgets' blue light emissions have the potential to inhibit melatonin production and make it difficult for you to fall asleep.

Watch Your Nutrition and Hydration: Since they might interfere with sleep patterns, big meals, coffee, nicotine, and alcohol should be avoided right before bed. Rather, choose small snacks when you're hungry and drink plenty of water during the day. However, avoid drinking too much in the hours before bed to reduce the number of times you wake up in the middle of the night to use the restroom.

Exercise Frequently: Physical activity during the day can help to improve the quality of your sleep. On the other hand, stay away from intense exercise right before bed as it could make you more alert and hinder your ability to go asleep.

Limit Daytime Naps: If you do take a nap during the day, try to limit it to no more than 20 to 30 minutes. Napping in the late afternoon or evening can make it difficult for you to fall asleep at night.

Handle Stress and Anxiety: Before going to bed, try some relaxation methods to assist soothe your body and mind, such as progressive muscle relaxation, deep breathing, or meditation. To help you decompress before bed, think about keeping a notebook where you may write down any worries or to-do lists.

Restrict Stimulants: Restrict your intake of stimulants like caffeine and nicotine, especially in the hours before bed. It may be more difficult to fall asleep and disturb sleep patterns after using these medications.

Seek Professional Assistance if Needed: You should think about speaking with a healthcare provider if, after following excellent sleep hygiene, you still have trouble falling asleep on a regular basis. They can assist in determining any underlying sleep disorders or other variables influencing your inability to sleep, as well as suggest the best course of action for therapy.

You may raise the quality of your sleep and enhance your general wellbeing by adopting these healthy sleep hygiene routines into your daily routine.

Controlling Anxiety and Stress

Improving sleep quality and general wellbeing requires effective stress and anxiety management. The following techniques will assist you in efficiently handling stress and anxiety:

Determine Triggers: Make a list of the events, ideas, or pursuits that usually set off your worry or tension. Being aware of these triggers might assist you in creating more efficient coping mechanisms.

Practice Relaxation Techniques: To assist calm your body and mind, incorporate relaxation techniques into your everyday routine. Effective techniques for lowering stress and fostering relaxation include gradual muscle relaxation, yoga, tai chi, deep breathing exercises, and meditation.

Exercise on a Regular Basis: Physical activity on a regular basis can assist lower stress and anxiety levels. On most days of the week, try to get in at least 30 minutes of moderate-intensity exercise. Pick enjoyable activities to engage in, like cycling, dancing, swimming, walking, or jogging.

Maintain a Healthy Lifestyle: Limit your intake of alcohol and caffeine, eat a balanced diet, and get enough sleep. These lifestyle choices may have an effect on your general wellbeing and stress levels.

Establish Boundaries: Develop the ability to decline assignments or obligations that will add to your stress or overwhelm. You can better manage your time and energy by setting up good boundaries.

Practice mindfulness: Mindfulness is accepting your thoughts and feelings without passing judgment on them and focusing on the here and now. You can increase your awareness and resilience to stresses by practicing mindfulness meditation and mindfulness-based stress reduction (MBSR) approaches.

Seek Support: Never be afraid to ask for help from friends, family, or a mental health professional. Speaking with reliable people about your emotions and experiences can be consoling and enlightening. Support groups, therapy, and counseling can all provide helpful direction and coping mechanisms.

Prioritize Self-Care: Give yourself the attention and time you deserve every day. Make time for the things that make you happy and relaxed, such reading a book, having a bath, listening to music, or going outside.

Develop a Gratitude Practice: Make a list of all the things you have each day to be grateful for. Reducing stress and changing your viewpoint can be achieved by concentrating on the positive aspects of your life.

Seek Professional Assistance if Necessary: If your attempts to manage your stress and anxiety are unsuccessful, you may want to consult a therapist, counselor, or psychiatrist. If required, they can offer tailored support, counseling, or medication.

You can learn useful techniques for handling stress and anxiety by applying these techniques into your daily routine. This will enhance your quality of life in terms of sleep, mental health, and general well-being.

CHAPTER THREE

Optimal Nutrition and Diet for Sleep

Enhancing nutrition and food can have a big impact on how well you sleep. Here are some food suggestions to encourage deeper sleep:

Aim for a diet that is well-balanced and has sufficient amounts of healthy fats, protein, and carbs. Foods high in protein include amino acids, which support neurotransmitter activity, and carbohydrates aid in the creation of serotonin, a neurotransmitter that controls sleep.

Select Complex Carbohydrates: Go for foods high in complex carbohydrates, like legumes, fruits, vegetables, and whole grains. These foods support blood sugar regulation and long-lasting energy, both of which can lead to more consistent sleep patterns.

Include Lean Proteins: Add low-fat dairy products, fish, chicken, tofu, beans, and lentils to your meals as lean protein sources. Tryptophan, an amino acid precursor to serotonin and melatonin, which are crucial for controlling sleep, is found in diets high in protein.

Limit Stimulants and Caffeine: Steer clear of or cut back on stimulants and caffeine, particularly in the afternoon and evening. By inhibiting adenosine, a neurotransmitter that encourages relaxation and drowsiness, caffeine can disrupt sleep.

Moderate Alcohol Consumption: Restrict your alcohol intake, particularly right before bed. Even though alcohol may make you feel drowsy at first, it might mess with your sleep cycles and cause you to sleep poorly or in pieces later in the evening.

Keep an Eye on Your Timing: Pay attention to when you consume your meals and snacks, particularly in regard to going to bed. Eat light or large meals several hours before going to bed to avoid pain and indigestion, which can make it difficult to fall asleep.

Keep Yourself Hydrated: To stay hydrated, drink lots of water throughout the day. However, avoid eating a lot of fluids right before bed to avoid having to wake up several times during the night to use the restroom.

Eat Foods Rich in Sleep-Supportive Nutrients: Include foods high in nutrients that promote restful sleep in your diet. For instance, meals high in magnesium, such as whole grains, nuts, and seeds, and leafy greens, might encourage relaxation and enhance the quality of sleep.

Think About Herbal Teas: As part of your nighttime routine, sip herbal teas like passionflower, valerian root, or chamomile. These teas offer ingredients that help induce calmness and sleep.

Listen to Your Body: Observe the effects of various foods and drinks on your sleep cycles.

Maintain a food journal to monitor your consumption and any variations in the length or quality of your sleep, then modify your diet as necessary.

You can optimize overall sleep quality and promote healthy sleep patterns by making thoughtful dietary and nutritional decisions. It's crucial to keep in mind that everyone reacts differently to diets, so experimenting with various meals and eating styles may be beneficial to determine what suits you the best. For individualized advice and assistance, think about speaking with a registered dietitian or other healthcare provider if you have particular worries about your food or sleep.

Including Exercise in Everyday Activities

Regular exercise can have a number of positive effects on your general wellbeing and quality of sleep. The following advice can help you include exercise to encourage deeper sleep:

Pick Pleasurable Activities: Opt for pleasurable and anticipated physical pursuits. Whether it's swimming, dancing, walking, jogging, cycling, or playing a sport, engaging in enjoyable and rewarding activities improves the likelihood that you'll continue with them over time.

Look for Opportunities to Move: Try to find ways to fit exercise into your everyday schedule. If at all feasible, walk or ride your bike to work, use the stairs rather than the elevator, and plan quick walks or stretching breaks throughout the day.

Establish Achievable Goals: When planning your workout, take into account your tastes, schedule, and current level of fitness. Over time, progressively increase the length, intensity, and frequency of your exercises by starting with simple, achievable goals.

Create a Regular Schedule: To create a routine, schedule your workouts for the same times every day. Exercise can be done consistently in the morning, during your lunch break, or in the evening to help you make it a regular part of your day.

Mix Up Your Workouts: To keep things fresh and avoid monotony, mix up your regimen by including a range of workouts and activities. Combine cardiovascular exercises with strength training, flexibility training, and leisure pursuits to engage diverse muscle groups and maintain a challenging physical environment.

Be Aware of Timing: Consider when you should exercise in relation to when you should sleep. While exercise might aid in improving sleep quality, for some persons it may have the opposite impact when done right before bed. To give your body enough time to wind down and relax, try to finish your workout a few hours before going to bed.

Listen to Your Body: Keep an eye on how exercise impacts your mood, energy level, and sleep schedule. While many people find that regular exercise helps them sleep better, other people may find that excessive or strenuous exercise, especially late in the day, interferes with their ability to sleep. Adapt your exercise regimen to your body's needs as it becomes apparent.

Practice Relaxation After Exercise: To assist your body and mind in settling into a state of relaxation, use relaxation techniques like deep breathing, yoga, or stretching after your workout. Better sleep can be encouraged by doing this, which can help offset any possible arousal effects of exercise.

Refuel and Stay Hydrated: To stay hydrated before and after exercise, drink lots of water. You should also refuel your body with wholesome foods to aid in healing and restore energy reserves.

Be Patient and Persistent: Getting the most out of exercise for sleep and general health requires consistency. Have patience with yourself, and don't give up if you don't see results right away or if you run into obstacles. Continue taking little, deliberate steps toward your goals.

Following these suggestions and adding regular exercise to your daily schedule will help you improve your general health and well-being, encourage better sleep, and reap the many advantages of leading an active lifestyle.

Tracking Development and Making Modifications

Optimizing sleep quality and resolving any potential problems require regular progress monitoring and habit modification. The following actions can help you keep an eye on your sleep and make any required adjustments:

Start with Recording Your Sleep: Track your sleeping habits, patterns, and any outside influences on your sleep by maintaining a sleep journal. Keep track of the times you go to bed and wake up, the length of time it takes you to fall asleep, the quality of your sleep, any nighttime awakenings, and your morning mood.

Employ Sleep Tracking Devices: To track your sleeping habits and collect information on the quality of your sleep, think about utilizing smartphone apps or sleep tracking devices. These gadgets can give you information on the length, quality, and cycles of your sleep as well as about your heart rate, breathing patterns, and movement while you're asleep.

Examine Sleep Environment: Make sure your sleeping environment is still restful by giving it a regular evaluation. To establish the ideal sleeping environment, check for elements like temperature, noise, light, and comfort level and make any necessary adjustments.

Evaluate Lifestyle Factors: Consider your lifestyle choices and how they might affect the quality of your sleep. Examine variables like alcohol and caffeine intake, physical activity routines, stress levels, screen time before bed, and nighttime rituals, and note any adjustments that might be required to enhance the quality of sleep.

Listen to Your Body: Observe how you feel during the day and how your sleep patterns impact your mood, energy, and general state of health. It can be an indication that you need to make changes to your sleep schedule if you are constantly feeling exhausted, agitated, or lethargic even though you are receiving enough sleep.

Find Patterns and Triggers: Keep an eye out for any patterns or situations that might be interfering with your sleep. Stress, anxiety, coffee, alcohol, inconsistent sleep cycles, and poor sleep hygiene practices are common factors. Making focused changes to enhance the quality of your sleep can be facilitated by recognizing these variables.

Modify Your Sleep Patterns Gradually: Modify your sleeping patterns methodically and gradually. Make gradual, doable adjustments at first, then track how they affect the quality of your sleep over time. This enables you to evaluate the effects of each modification and make more improvements as necessary.

Seek Professional Assistance if Needed: You should think about consulting a healthcare provider or sleep specialist if, despite changing your sleeping patterns, you are still having trouble falling asleep. In addition to offering individualized recommendations and treatment alternatives catered to your specific needs, they can assist in identifying underlying concerns.

Be Patient and Persistent: It frequently takes patience and persistence to improve sleep habits and treat sleep-related disorders. While you strive to make positive adjustments, practice self-compassion and don't give up if you don't see results right away. Remain dedicated to putting a high priority on proper sleep hygiene and adapting as necessary to promote better sleep.

You may gradually improve the quality of your sleep and your general well-being by keeping an eye on your sleep patterns, assessing your sleeping environment and habits, and making focused changes as needed.

CONCLUSION

treating sleep issues calls for a diversified strategy that takes into account a range of environmental, behavioral, and lifestyle variables. People can take proactive measures to maximize their overall well-being and quality of sleep by including regular exercise, managing stress and anxiety, improving sleep hygiene, and making modifications based on progress monitoring.

Important things to think about when treating sleep issues are as follows:

Identifying Sleep Problems: In order to seek the right interventions, it is critical to recognize common sleep concerns such as insomnia, sleep apnea, restless legs syndrome, or circadian rhythm disturbances.

Enhancing Sleep Hygiene: You can improve the quality of your sleep by practicing relaxation techniques before bed, keeping a regular sleep schedule, and designing a sleep-friendly atmosphere.

Handling Stress and Anxiety: Using stress-reduction strategies including regular exercise, deep breathing, and mindfulness can help reduce psychological issues that lead to sleep problems.

Exercise: Frequent physical activity, with consideration for time and intensity, can improve sleep quality and foster calm.

Tracking Development and Making Modifications: People can find trends, triggers, and opportunities for development by keeping an eye on their sleep schedule, way of life, and surroundings. Refining sleep habits and addressing chronic difficulties can be accomplished by making progressive improvements based on progress monitoring.

Seeking Professional Assistance When Necessary: Getting in touch with medical experts, such therapists or sleep specialists, can offer individualized advice, diagnostic testing, and treatment choices for resolving underlying sleep disorders or chronic sleep issues.

general, people can improve their general health and well-being, get better quality sleep, and get the advantages of peaceful, revitalizing sleep by tackling sleep issues proactively and holistically.

THE END